FROM MANAGING TO CONQUERING VAGINAL CANCER

Expert Guide To Understanding The Causes, Recognizing Symptoms, And Navigating Treatment For A Path To Healthy Living

DR. DASHIELL DANIEL

"Vaginal Cancer" is a comprehensive and valuable resource in the field of oncology, addressing a critical element of women's health that is often overlooked. The importance of this work is highlighted by its comprehensive investigation of the numerous characteristics of vaginal cancer, from recognizing its various forms and subtypes to illuminating the delicate processes of diagnosis, staging, and treatment. In their pursuit of scholarly excellence, the writers offer readers a nuanced viewpoint on the causes, risk factors, signs, and symptoms of this type of cancer, creating a thorough awareness of the disease.

The book's commitment to holistic patient care is obvious in the extensive analysis of coping techniques, emotional effects, and support systems accessible to people diagnosed with vaginal cancer. The inclusion of chapters on survivorship, follow-up care, and preventative strategies provides a practical dimension to the book, providing useful insights into life after treatment and fighting for women's health.

The authors discuss not only medical interventions like surgery, radiation therapy, chemotherapy, targeted therapy, and immunotherapy but also the importance of emotional well-being and maintaining a high quality of life throughout the journey. The book goes beyond a professional approach by including success stories and inspirational experiences, giving readers hope and empowerment.

This academic tome not only adds to the medical literature on gynecological oncology, but also serves as a lighthouse for anyone looking for in-depth information about vaginal cancer. By delving into the complexities of this complex disease, the book emerges as a crucial tool for healthcare professionals, academics, and advocates alike, encouraging a broader conversation on women's health and building compassion for people afflicted by vaginal cancer.

Introduction

Vaginal cancer, an uncommon but dangerous kind of cancer, offers major health risks to women.

This book attempts to provide a thorough examination of the numerous facets of overcoming vaginal cancer, giving light on the complexities of its diagnosis, treatment, and prevention. We hope to contribute to a greater understanding of vaginal cancer and empower individuals with knowledge that can lead to better results by digging into its scientific, medical, and societal elements.

The Goal Of The Book

The major goal of this book is to serve as an authoritative and informative resource for those affected by vaginal cancer, their families, healthcare professionals, and the larger community. The book strives to raise awareness, promote early detection, and demystify the difficulties of vaginal cancer through an in-depth assessment of the present state of knowledge, emerging research, and breakthroughs in medical technologies.

We believe that by providing a nuanced perspective, we may bridge the gap between scientific facts and practical insights, giving readers the skills they need to handle the obstacles associated with this disease.

Personal Relationship To The Subject

The author's connection to the subject was a driving force in the creation of this work.

Whether via personal experience with vaginal cancer or a deep empathy for those who have encountered this illness, the contributors are united in their desire to make a positive difference in the lives of those touched by this disease. We hope to personalize the path of people dealing with vaginal cancer by weaving personal narratives into the fabric of scientific inquiry, creating a holistic knowledge that goes beyond clinical numbers and medical language.

The Value Of Addressing Vaginal Cancer

Beyond the statistical rarity of vaginal cancer, addressing it is critical. Despite having a lower frequency than other gynecological cancers, vaginal cancer has a significant impact on afflicted individuals and their communities.

The physical and mental toll, combined with the possibility of considerable morbidity and mortality, emphasizes the importance of coordinated efforts to confront and fight this condition.

Understanding the socio-cultural factors that contribute to delayed diagnosis and limited access to care is also important for establishing effective ways to lessen the burden of vaginal cancer on disadvantaged communities.

Vaginal Cancer Diagnosis

Accurate and prompt detection is critical in the fight against vaginal cancer. A medical history evaluation, physical examination, imaging investigations, and biopsy are all part of the diagnosis process. This book delves into the subtleties of each diagnostic modality, examining its strengths and limits as well as the expanding landscape of novel diagnostic techniques.

The importance of early detection will be emphasized, as will the responsibility of healthcare practitioners in raising awareness, routine screenings, and rapid follow-up for persons at risk or presenting suspected symptoms.

Prognosis And Staging

The importance of staging in detecting the degree of vaginal cancer and guiding treatment decisions cannot be overstated. This chapter will thoroughly examine the various staging systems used in clinical practice, evaluating their importance, evolution, and impact on prognosis.

Furthermore, insights into prognostic markers such as tumor features, lymph node involvement, and the occurrence of distant metastases will be provided. A sophisticated grasp of the prognostic picture is required for customizing treatment strategies and encouraging informed interactions between healthcare providers and patients.

Treatment Options

Vaginal cancer treatment is diverse, comprising surgery, radiation therapy, chemotherapy, and developing targeted medicines. This section will go over each therapy method in detail, looking at their mechanisms of action, indications, and potential adverse effects. The expanding subject of personalized medicine, in which the identification of specific molecular targets allows for specialized therapeutic methods, will receive special focus. The difficulties of reconciling efficacy with quality-of-life concerns will be explored, highlighting the significance of a multidisciplinary approach to optimizing patient outcomes.

Surgical Procedures

Surgery plays an important part in the treatment of vaginal cancer, from local excision for early-stage illness to more extensive treatments for advanced instances. This section will go over the various surgical procedures, such as radical surgery, lymphadenectomy, and reconstructive operations. The intricacies of minimally invasive procedures and their impact on postoperative recovery will be investigated, as will fertility preservation considerations and the psychosocial implications of surgical operations.

This book seeks to give individuals and healthcare practitioners the knowledge they need to make informed decisions about the best treatment method by conducting a thorough evaluation of surgical possibilities.

Radiation Treatment

Radiation therapy is an important component in the treatment of vaginal cancer, whether as a primary treatment modality or as part of a multimodal approach. This section will go over the many methods of radiation therapy, including external beam radiation and brachytherapy.

Treatment planning, dose escalation, and the expanding importance of modern technologies like intensity-modulated radiation therapy (IMRT) and proton therapy will be covered.

Furthermore, insights into the potential long-term effects of radiation will be addressed, as will techniques for reducing treatment-related problems to improve the overall quality of care for persons undergoing radiation therapy.

Systemic Therapies And Chemotherapy

Chemotherapy, both as a stand-alone treatment and in conjunction with other modalities, is critical in the treatment of vaginal cancer.

This part will go over the numerous chemotherapy medicines, their modes of action, and their specific applications in various stages of the disease. Furthermore, the developing landscape of targeted treatments and immunotherapies will be investigated, emphasizing their potential for enhancing treatment results and decreasing systemic adverse effects. A thorough grasp of systemic medicines is required for designing treatment regimens, controlling side effects, and optimizing therapeutic benefits for women with vaginal cancer.

Aftercare And Survivorship

The road to recovery from vaginal cancer does not end with the conclusion of initial treatment, stressing the significance of long-term follow-up care and survivability.

This section will look at the problems and opportunities that come with being a survivor, focusing on the physical, emotional, and psychosocial elements of healing. The role of surveillance measures in monitoring for recurrence, including imaging scans and biomarkers, will be emphasized. In addition, survivors and healthcare practitioners will be given insights into the expanding landscape of survivorship care plans, rehabilitation, and support services to help them navigate the post-treatment part of the cancer journey.

Early Detection And Prevention

Early detection and prevention are critical components of a complete strategy to defeat vaginal cancer. This section will look at primary prevention strategies, such as immunization against the human papillomavirus (HPV), which is a key risk factor for vaginal cancer.

The role of lifestyle changes in lowering the risk of vaginal cancer, such as smoking cessation and safe sexual practices, will be explored. The need for early detection will also be stressed through routine screenings, awareness campaigns, and education. This book aims to empower people and communities in preventing vaginal cancer by addressing modifiable risk factors and advocating proactive health behaviors.

Considerations From A Socio-Cultural Perspective

Due to socio-cultural factors that influence access to healthcare, health-seeking habits, and overall health outcomes, certain populations are disproportionately affected by vaginal cancer.

This section will critically analyze these aspects, such as healthcare access discrepancies, cultural taboos around gynecological health, and the impact of socioeconomic position on cancer outcomes. Strategies for increasing health equity, culturally competent healthcare, and community participation will be investigated.

This book intends to contribute to a more inclusive and equitable strategy for overcoming vaginal cancer by considering socio-cultural concerns, ensuring that all individuals have access to timely and appropriate care.

New Research And Innovations

The field of vaginal cancer research is dynamic, with continual advances in understanding the disease's molecular foundation and investigating novel treatment approaches. This section will provide an overview of cutting-edge research, such as genetic studies, immunotherapy trials, and novel diagnostic methods. Artificial intelligence's potential impact on cancer detection and individualized treatment planning will be investigated. Healthcare practitioners, researchers, and individuals affected by vaginal cancer can contribute to and benefit from the developing landscape of cancer care by remaining current on novel research and technologies.

overcoming vaginal cancer necessitates a holistic approach that includes early identification, customized treatment options, survivorship care, and a commitment to tackling socio-cultural issues that contribute to health inequities.

This book intends to be a comprehensive resource for people navigating the intricacies of vaginal cancer, including information from diagnosis to survivorship. We hope to contribute to the collaborative effort to overcome the problems faced by vaginal cancer and enhance the lives of women afflicted by this disease by combining scientific rigor with personal narratives and a focus on health justice.

CHAPTER ONE
UNDERSTANDING VAGINAL CANCER

Vaginal cancer is an uncommon and sometimes misdiagnosed kind of gynecological cancer that develops in the cells of the vagina, the muscular tube that connects the uterus to the external genitals. Despite its rarity in comparison to other gynecological malignancies, it remains a major public health concern because of the potential impact on women's reproductive and general health.

This syndrome develops when normal cells in the vagina experience aberrant alterations, resulting in uncontrolled proliferation and tumor formation. Vaginal cancer is divided into several categories and subtypes, each with its own set of characteristics and implications for diagnosis and treatment.

Subtypes And Types

Squamous Cell Carcinoma Squamous cell carcinoma is the most prevalent type of vaginal cancer, and it begins in the thin, flat cells that line the vaginal surface. These cells become cancerous, and the ensuing tumors can damage various areas of the vagina. Squamous cell cancer is frequently related to persistent human papillomavirus (HPV) infection, highlighting the necessity of HPV vaccination and regular screenings.

Adenocarcinoma develops in the glandular cells that create mucus and other fluids in the vagina. This kind of cancer is less prevalent than squamous cell carcinoma, but it presents unique diagnostic and therapy issues. Adenocarcinoma can develop in a variety of locations within the vagina, including the upper section near the cervix. Understanding the unique features of adenocarcinoma is critical for developing effective therapeutic methods.

Clear Cell Carcinoma is an uncommon subtype of vaginal cancer that frequently appears in women who were exposed to diethylstilboestrol (DES) during fetal development. Between the 1940s and the 1970s, pregnant women were given DES, a synthetic estrogen. Because of its relationship with DES exposure, clear cell carcinoma presents unique diagnostic and therapeutic problems, necessitating a sophisticated approach to patient treatment.

Other unusual kinds Aside from the more common kinds discussed above, there are some unusual subtypes of vaginal cancer. Sarcomas, melanomas, and various histological variations are examples. While these unusual varieties account for a lesser proportion of all occurrences, their distinct characteristics demand specialist diagnostic procedures and treatment options. Understanding these unusual subgroups in depth is critical for giving accurate prognoses and enhancing patient outcomes.

Factors Of Risk And Causes

The etiology of vaginal cancer is complex, encompassing genetic, environmental, and lifestyle factors. Persistent infection with high-risk HPV strains is a major risk factor, especially for squamous cell carcinoma. HPV vaccination has emerged as an important preventive measure, helping to reduce the prevalence of HPV-related malignancies such as vaginal cancer. A history of cervical cancer, smoking, age, DES exposure, and certain genetic disorders are all risk factors. Investigating the interactions of these factors can help in the prevention and early identification of vaginal cancer.

Symptoms And Signs

Recognizing the signs and symptoms of vaginal cancer is critical for early detection and treatment. Abnormal vaginal bleeding, pain during sexual intercourse, pelvic pain, and changes in vaginal discharge are all common signs. These symptoms, however, are generic and might be related to a variety of gynecological disorders. As a result, healthcare providers must distinguish vaginal cancer from other benign or malignant illnesses. Setting specific diagnostic criteria and applying modern imaging techniques can improve diagnostic accuracy and permit quick action.

Finally, a thorough study of vaginal cancer includes its definition, categorization into categories and subtypes, investigation of causes and risk factors, and identification of signs and symptoms. Each aspect of this knowledge is critical for healthcare workers involved in vaginal cancer prevention, diagnosis, and therapy.

As research advances, continuous attempts to expand our understanding of this condition will contribute to better outcomes for affected individuals, underlining the significance of a multidisciplinary approach to vaginal cancer treatment.

CHAPTER TWO
DIAGNOSIS AND STAGING

Early detection methods are critical for successful vaginal cancer management. The Pap smear, a widely used procedure that includes collecting cells from the cervix and vagina to determine any abnormalities, is one of the key screening tools for early detection. Furthermore, human papillomavirus (HPV) testing is frequently paired with Pap smears to improve sensitivity. HPV, particularly high-risk strains, is a substantial risk factor for vaginal cancer. These screening procedures aid in the detection of precancerous lesions, allowing for timely intervention and lowering the risk of disease progression.

Biopsies are required to confirm a diagnosis of vaginal cancer. Following a bad Pap smear or HPV test results, a biopsy is performed to acquire tissue samples from the afflicted area. This enables for a thorough evaluation of the cellular composition, which aids in evaluating the type, grade, and extent of invasion of the cancer. Depending on the presumed location and size of the lesion, different biopsy procedures, such as colposcopy-guided biopsy or cone biopsy, may be used. The results of biopsies are critical in making an accurate diagnosis and developing an appropriate treatment plan.

Imaging studies, in addition to these direct diagnostic approaches, are critical in determining the degree and features of vaginal cancer. Magnetic Resonance Imaging (MRI) is a non-invasive imaging procedure that produces precise images of the pelvic region, allowing doctors to see tumor size, location, and potential invasion into surrounding structures. CT scans, which provide cross-sectional images of the pelvic area, are very useful in determining the spread of cancer. Positron Emission Tomography (PET) scans can detect metastases by identifying aberrant metabolic activity in distant organs. These imaging modalities work together to provide a thorough understanding of the condition and guide therapy decisions.

The staging method is critical in evaluating the amount of vaginal cancer and in developing a suitable treatment strategy. The International Federation of Gynecology and Obstetrics (FIGO) staging system is commonly used to classify cancer severity based on characteristics such as tumor size, involvement of neighboring tissues, and lymph node status. This approach aids in the classification of disease phases, which range from early stages with localized tumors to advanced stages with regional or distant spread.

The TNM staging approach, which takes into account the size and extent of the primary tumor (T), the involvement of regional lymph nodes (N), and the occurrence of distant metastasis (M), adds to the staging procedure. These staging systems work together to standardize the assessment of vaginal cancer, improve communication among healthcare practitioners, and guide treatment options.

diagnosing and staging vaginal cancer requires a multifaceted strategy that includes early detection approaches, biopsy procedures, and modern imaging techniques. The combination of Pap smears and HPV testing identifies precancerous lesions, while biopsy techniques confirm the diagnosis and give critical information for treatment planning. Imaging examinations, including MRI, CT scans, and PET scans, help to provide a complete picture of the condition. The staging approach, which employs systems such as FIGO and TNM, improves our awareness of the amount of vaginal cancer and assists healthcare providers in developing appropriate treatment plans.

This comprehensive diagnostic and staging strategy is critical for improving patient outcomes and creating a more precise and tailored approach to vaginal cancer care.

CHAPTER THREE
TREATMENT OPTIONS

Vaginal cancer is a very uncommon disease that affects the cells that line the vagina. Vaginal cancer treatment is interdisciplinary, with many techniques aimed at eradicating or controlling the illness. Surgery is the main therapeutic option for vaginal cancer and is crucial in its management.

A frequent treatment is radical hysterectomy, which involves the removal of the uterus, surrounding tissues, and the upper section of the vagina. When the cancer is restricted to the upper region of the vagina or includes the cervix, this major surgery is frequently performed.

Pelvic exenteration is a much more invasive surgical procedure. The whole pelvic organs, including the bladder, rectum, and sections of the colon, as well as the uterus and vagina, are removed during this treatment. Pelvic exenteration is usually reserved for advanced vaginal cancer that has progressed throughout the pelvic cavity. In carefully selected individuals, pelvic exenteration can give a prospect of cure or long-term illness control despite its harsh nature.

Radiation therapy, in addition to surgery, is an important component of the treatment arsenal for vaginal cancer. External beam radiation is delivered from outside the body and focuses on malignant tissues. This method is frequently used after surgery to eradicate any remaining cancer cells and lower the chance of recurrence.

Another type of radiation therapy is brachytherapy, which involves inserting radioactive sources directly into or around the tumor. Brachytherapy is widely utilized to address residual illness or as a primary therapeutic strategy in the setting of vaginal cancer.

Chemotherapy, a systemic treatment that uses medications to eliminate or inhibit the growth of cancer cells, is commonly used to treat vaginal cancer. This method is especially useful when the cancer has gone beyond the boundaries of the vagina or when surgery and radiation alone may not be enough. Chemotherapy medications can be taken orally or intravenously and circulate throughout the body, targeting cancer cells both locally and distantly.

Targeted therapy is a relatively new treatment option for vaginal cancer. This method employs medications that selectively target certain chemicals involved in cancer cell growth and survival. Targeted therapy, by focusing on these specific targets, can be more precise and perhaps cause fewer side effects than standard chemotherapy.

The discovery of unique molecular markers in vaginal cancer has paved the path for the development of targeted medicines, allowing for a more personalized and effective treatment approach.

Immunotherapy is a novel and fast-expanding field in the treatment of cancer, especially vaginal cancer.

This method uses the body's immune system to identify and eliminate cancer cells. Immunotherapy medications, such as immune checkpoint inhibitors, have shown promise in the treatment of many malignancies by allowing the immune system to assault cancer cells.

While research into immunotherapy for vaginal cancer is ongoing, preliminary findings suggest that it could be a valuable addition to the therapeutic arsenal, particularly in cases where previous treatments have proven ineffective.

Finally, the treatment of vaginal cancer requires a comprehensive and integrated approach, with specific roles for surgery, radiation therapy, chemotherapy, targeted therapy, and immunotherapy. The treatment techniques used are determined by several criteria, including the stage of the cancer, the extent of metastasis, and the patient's overall condition.

A multidisciplinary team of surgeons, radiation oncologists, medical oncologists, and other specialists works together to create a treatment plan that maximizes the odds of success while minimizing the impact on the patient's quality of life. As research advances, the landscape of vaginal cancer treatment options is set to change, providing fresh hope and better outcomes for those facing this difficult diagnosis.

CHAPTER FOUR
COPING WITH VAGINAL CANCER

Vaginal cancer is a difficult diagnosis that not only impacts an individual's physical health but also has a significant emotional impact. The emotional toll of being diagnosed with cancer cannot be understated. Fear, worry, despair, and concern about the future are common emotions experienced by patients. Because of the personal nature of the affected area, the emotional impact of vaginal cancer can be extremely difficult. Patients may struggle with body image, self-esteem, and sexuality concerns. The emotional side of vaginal cancer must be addressed for a comprehensive approach to therapy and recovery.

System of Support

Building and maintaining a strong support network is critical for people dealing with vaginal cancer. During difficult times, family and friends play an important role in offering emotional support, practical assistance, and a sense of normalcy.

The involvement of loved ones can considerably improve patients' well-being by assisting them in coping with the mental and physical obstacles connected with cancer. The unwavering support of family and friends provides a sense of belonging and can improve the overall mental health of women confronting vaginal cancer.

Groups Of Support

In addition to familial support, participation in support groups can be a unique and significant resource for women with vaginal cancer. Support groups allow patients to connect with others who have had similar experiences, establishing a community where people can openly communicate their concerns, anxieties, and accomplishments. Peer support can be empowering since it can provide insights into coping tactics, therapeutic experiences, and long-term survival. These groups promote a sense of community, lowering feelings of isolation and assisting patients in developing resilience in the face of hardship.

Assistance With Counseling

Professional counseling services are critical in dealing with the psychological effects of vaginal cancer. Oncology-trained counselors can provide patients with specialized emotional support, aiding them in navigating the complicated emotional terrain that comes with a cancer diagnosis. Counseling sessions may include discussions about coping skills, stress management, and strategies for maintaining a positive attitude throughout the treatment process.

The incorporation of counseling services into the entire care plan contributes to the holistic well-being of vaginal cancer patients.

Maintaining Life Quality

Maintaining a high quality of life becomes a primary emphasis of comprehensive care as patients face the challenges of vaginal cancer. This entails not only addressing the physical components of health but also the larger dimensions that contribute to overall well-being.

Nutrition

Nutrition is critical to the health and recovery of people suffering from vaginal cancer. A nutritious and well-balanced diet is crucial for boosting the immune system, increasing energy levels, and aiding in the healing process. Oncology nutritionists assist patients in creating individualized dietary programs that address particular nutritional demands while mitigating the potential negative effects of cancer therapy. Stressing the importance of diet is critical to improving the overall health and resilience of women confronting vaginal cancer.

Exercise

Physical activity is essential for people with vaginal cancer to maintain their quality of life.

Exercise has been demonstrated to increase physical function, reduce weariness, and improve mental health. Tailored fitness regimens, developed in collaboration with healthcare specialists, take into account the specific demands and limits of cancer patients. Exercise not only improves patients' physical strength but also works as a stress reliever and a technique for creating a positive body image.

Integrative Medicine

Complementary and integrative therapies have emerged as effective supplements to standard cancer care. These therapies, which include acupuncture, yoga, and meditation, are intended to improve the general well-being of people dealing with vaginal cancer. Integrative treatments address patients' entire needs, including physical, emotional, and spiritual aspects. Integrative therapies are frequently incorporated into treatment plans to assist patients with additional skills for coping with cancer problems, increasing relaxation, and enhancing overall quality of life.

beating vaginal cancer necessitates a multifaceted approach that goes beyond medical interventions. A holistic care plan includes coping with the emotional effect, developing a strong support system, and focusing on maintaining quality of life through nutrition, exercise, and integrative therapies. Individuals experiencing vaginal cancer can improve their overall well-being and resilience by addressing the physical, emotional, and lifestyle components of the cancer experience, paving the way for recovery and long-term health.

CHAPTER FIVE
SURVIVORSHIP AND AFTERCARE

Survivorship in the context of overcoming vaginal cancer denotes a vital phase in the continuum of care, representing the time after the main therapy is completed. This phase encompasses a multidimensional strategy that goes beyond physical healing to include psychological, emotional, and social aspects. The survivorship journey demonstrates the strength of those who have endured the trials of vaginal cancer. It is critical for healthcare practitioners to develop complete survivorship care plans, ensuring that survivors have the tools they need to negotiate the complexities of life after treatment.

<u>Following Treatment:</u>

Life after vaginal cancer treatment is a difficult terrain in which survivors must make both physical and emotional adjustments.

Physical healing includes dealing with difficulties such as weariness, soreness, and possibly changes in sexual function. Survivors may also need to re-establish a feeling of normalcy in their everyday lives, such as returning to work, managing relationships, and revising personal goals.

A comprehensive approach to life following treatment includes rehabilitation programs, survivorship clinics, and support groups, all of which contribute to survivors' overall well-being.

By addressing these issues, healthcare providers can help survivors embrace life after cancer.

<u>Recurrence monitoring:</u>

In the post-treatment phase of vaginal cancer, vigilant monitoring for recurrence is critical.

Given the possibility of cancer recurrence, regular follow-up checkups and surveillance are critical components of survivorship care. To detect early indicators of recurrence, healthcare providers use a combination of imaging scans, laboratory tests, and clinical evaluations.

Effective communication between healthcare providers and survivors is critical because it allows for the early identification of symptoms and concerns, allowing for prompt action if necessary. Monitoring for recurrence includes not just the medical issues, but also addressing the emotional toll that survivors may experience as a result of the anxiety of recurrence.

<u>Long-Term Adverse Effects:</u>

Long-term adverse effects of vaginal cancer treatment are a delicate component of survival that requires close monitoring. While radiation therapy and chemotherapy are critical in the elimination of cancer cells, they may cause long-term adverse effects that damage the survivor's quality of life. These can take the form of persistent discomfort, infertility concerns, or changes in bowel and bladder function. Recognizing and managing these long-term negative effects would necessitate a coordinated effort on the part of healthcare practitioners and survivors. Rehabilitation programs, targeted interventions, and continuing support are critical components in reducing the impact of long-term side effects and promoting a more favorable post-treatment trajectory.

Emotional And Psychological Health

The emotional and psychological well-being of survivors following vaginal cancer therapy is an important component of comprehensive care.

The emotional toll of cancer, along with the fear of recurrence, needs a supportive environment that recognizes the psychosocial issues survivors encounter. Counseling and psychotherapy, among other mental health interventions, are critical in addressing anxiety, sadness, and post-traumatic stress disorder that may accompany the survivorship journey. Furthermore, support groups and survival clinics allow survivors to connect, exchange stories, and gain strength from a shared understanding. Recognizing and addressing survivorship's emotional and psychological components is critical to creating resilience and maintaining a good attitude toward life after cancer.

overcoming vaginal cancer necessitates a continuum of care that extends far beyond the completion of the first treatment.

Physical recovery, continuous monitoring for recurrence, management of long-term side effects, and addressing survivors' emotional and psychological well-being are all aspects of survivor care. Healthcare practitioners can assist survivors to negotiate the complexity of life after vaginal cancer by using a thorough and patient-centered approach, developing resilience and promoting a holistic sense of well-being.

CHAPTER SIX
PREVENTION AND ADVOCACY

Vaginal cancer is a major health risk for women all over the world, making prevention and advocacy critical components of a holistic healthcare plan. Human Papillomavirus (HPV) immunizations are an important part of prevention. HPV is a well-known risk factor for vaginal cancer, and vaccines targeting specific HPV strains have been shown to reduce the prevalence of infections that can lead to cancer. Healthcare institutions can make significant progress in reducing vaginal cancer and its effects by lobbying for widespread HPV vaccination.

Regular screening and check-ups are critical in detecting and preventing vaginal cancer. Routine gynecological exams, including as Pap smears and HPV tests, allow healthcare providers to detect precancerous lesions or early-stage malignancies. Early identification improves treatment outcomes and lowers mortality rates in women with vaginal cancer. In the context of preventing and managing vaginal cancer, promoting regular screenings and check-ups as part of women's healthcare routines becomes critical.

Advocating for women's health is a holistic approach that includes factors other than cancer prevention. Advocating for women's health entails supporting comprehensive healthcare, such as access to reproductive health services, family planning, and education on lifestyle issues that affect general well-being. Communities and legislators may establish an environment that supports both prevention and effective management of vaginal cancer by addressing the broader range of women's health.

Raising awareness is an important tactic in the fight against vaginal cancer since an informed population is more likely to take preventive measures and seek timely medical assistance. Information on risk factors, symptoms, and the necessity of early detection should be disseminated through public awareness programs. Furthermore, these initiatives can assist in dispelling misunderstandings and stigmas associated with vaginal cancer, building a supportive atmosphere for individuals afflicted, and encouraging open talks about women's health.

Research funding is critical for furthering our understanding of vaginal cancer, establishing novel preventative techniques, and improving treatment options. Research efforts should concentrate on finding additional risk factors, improving screening procedures, and investigating novel therapy options. By investing in scientific research, healthcare systems can continuously improve their approaches to vaginal cancer prevention and treatment, thereby minimizing the disease's impact on individuals and society.

Finally, overcoming vaginal cancer necessitates a thorough and coordinated effort focusing on prevention and advocacy.

Each notion is important in minimizing the incidence and effect of vaginal cancer, from supporting HPV vaccination and frequent screenings to campaigning for women's health and raising awareness. Furthermore, funding research keeps our strategies at the forefront of scientific developments. We may work toward a future where vaginal cancer is a preventable and manageable health concern by incorporating these ideas into healthcare legislation and community efforts.

CHAPTER SEVEN

INSPIRATIONAL JOURNEYS AND SUCCESS STORIES

Individuals who have successfully overcome vaginal cancer frequently share their personal stories as a source of motivation for others experiencing similar struggles. These stories highlight survivors' fortitude and courage, revealing the mental and physical challenges they faced along the way. Personal accounts offer light on the many facets of battling vaginal cancer, such as the initial diagnosis, various treatment options, and the post-therapy phase. Survivors frequently underline the significance of maintaining a positive attitude, having a strong support system, and relying on healthcare professionals to help them recover. These stories not only give people hope, but they also help to raise awareness about vaginal cancer and the need for early identification and intervention.

Overcoming Obstacles: The battle against vaginal cancer is fraught with numerous physical and mental obstacles. Patients must navigate complicated treatment regimens, which may involve surgery, chemotherapy, and radiation therapy. These therapies' adverse effects can be physically and emotionally draining, lowering one's overall quality of life. Overcoming obstacles include not just dealing with the acute effects of cancer, but also dealing with long-term consequences such as fertility troubles, sexual dysfunction, and psychological distress. Patients frequently work with interdisciplinary healthcare teams, including oncologists, psychiatrists, and rehabilitation specialists, to establish tailored strategies for dealing with these difficulties. Understanding and overcoming the numerous hurdles experienced during treatment are critical components of overcoming vaginal cancer.

Survivors of vaginal cancer play an important role in empowering others who are dealing with the disease.

Their stories serve as a light of hope for those who are presently undergoing treatment or have recently been diagnosed. Advocacy, support groups, and educational activities are all forms of empowerment that go beyond personal tales. Survivors are frequently turned into champions for early identification and prevention, taking part in awareness campaigns and fundraising activities. Support groups give a forum for survivors to interact, exchange stories, and offer advice to those facing similar challenges.

Survivors often participate in educational projects aimed at dispelling stereotypes about vaginal cancer, encouraging frequent screenings, and encouraging a proactive approach to women's health. Individual stories, community engagement, and a desire to increase general awareness and outcomes all contribute to the empowerment of others in the context of vaginal cancer.

CONCLUSION

overcoming vaginal cancer is a complicated process that includes personal achievements, overcoming huge hurdles, and empowering others in the community. Success tales of women who have confronted and overcome vaginal cancer serve as strong testaments to the human spirit's tenacity. These stories offer important insights into the various stages of the cancer journey, from diagnosis to treatment and recovery. Overcoming the physical and emotional tolls of cancer treatment necessitates a multifaceted approach that includes not just medical interventions but also psychological and social support.

The empowerment of others is a natural continuation of the survivor's journey, as they contribute to vaginal cancer awareness, advocacy, and support networks.

In the face of vaginal cancer, the collective influence of personal achievements, conquering hurdles, and encouraging others results in a more knowledgeable and resilient community.

The panorama of vaginal cancer is steadily shifting as medical advances continue to evolve and awareness efforts gain traction. Early detection, better treatment options, and a comprehensive approach to patient care all lead to better outcomes. The win over vaginal cancer, however, is more than a medical achievement; it is a monument to the fortitude, commitment, and collaborative efforts of survivors, healthcare professionals, and support networks. Success in the fight against vaginal cancer is measured not only by remission, but also by the lasting impact survivors have on others and the beneficial improvements they bring to the greater landscape of women's health.

9 798872 469131